NEVER
BRUSH
YOUR TEETH
AGAIN!

NEVER BRUSH YOUR TEETH AGAIN!

STARTLING INFORMATION ON HOW ORAL HEALTH IMPACTS YOUR ENTIRE BODY

BY P., PIERO DDS

Universal Wellness Publication
2014

Never Brush Your Teeth Again!
Copyright © 2014 P., Piero DDS

To promote health world-wide, anything in this book may
be reproduced and used PROVIDING the following is
included: "Reproduced from Never Brush Your Teeth
Again! written by P., Piero DDS"

Universal Wellness Publication
info@dentalairforce.com

ISBN-13: 978-1503321083
ISBN-10: 1503321088

Contents

Introduction

This is not a book with happy drawings of smiling teeth holding hands with a toothbrush. To be perfectly frank, the toothbrush and teeth are not good companions. Toothbrushes damage tooth enamel and score the root base of teeth through over-abrasion. On top of that, they do a poor job of removing the biofilm, bacteria, viruses, and worm-like creatures living in, on, and around your teeth. With only a 30 percent efficacy rate, the toothbrush should have been fired from its job long ago.

Within these pages you are going to learn about the scary things in your mouth that could literally kill you—a bio-system of bacteria, yeast, and viruses so aggressive it can reproduce by the billions within a few hours of traditional brushing. These unwelcome parasites cause periodontal disease and contribute to many deadly health problems, such as diabetes, heart disease, COPD, arthritis, and many cancers.

The information presented is based on clinical international medical and dental research studies reported by the Centers for Disease Control, the National Institute of Health, and articles appearing in professional peer-reviewed health and dental publications, including:

- *Journal of the American Dental Association*
- *Journal of Periodontology*
- *Journal of Clinical Periodontology*
- *Journal of Public Health Dentistry*
- *Journal of Clinical Pediatric Dentistry*
- *International Journal of Experimental Dental Science*

A list of citations for personal review is available in the References section.

Never Brush Your Teeth Again! will also introduce the public and dentists to a remarkable solution to these threats—Dental Air Force. This daily home oral cleaning system (cleared by the FDA for marketing), removes plaque, biofilm, germs, and bacteria from your teeth and protects people from periodontal disease and associated illnesses far more effectively than brushing and oral irrigating.

In fact, I sincerely hope this book raises your awareness to the point where you are convinced to throw away your manual or electric toothbrush and replace them with Dental Air Force that will, in the long run, save you and your family thousands of dollars in dental bills and improve your health, quality of life, and longevity.

Chapter 1

The Zoo in Your Mouth

Your mouth is like a microbiological zoo, comprised of more than 700 different species of bacteria, yeast, viruses, and flagellate worm-like mobile creatures called spirochetes. [Ref 1]

These species are divided into two different groups, aerobic and anaerobic—fancy words describing the kind of bacteria that flourish in the presence of air (aerobic), or the kind that breed and thrive in the absence of air (anaerobic).

Some of these bugs are beneficial, but many are contagious, smelly, infectious, and invasive. They can be described as imbedding, twisted, carnivorous, opportunistic, greasy, and/or acidic.

More bacteria live in your mouth right now than people on the planet—between 30 billion and 100 billion "bugs." The anaerobic bacteria living deep in the biofilm on your teeth feed not only on the carbohydrates you consume, but also on protein from sloughing tissue, dead and dying cells, and blood.

We are not born with these organisms. We are exposed to them by our interactions, environment, what we eat, and even the air we breathe. Where we live, how we live, where we travel, how often we wash our hands, whom we kiss, what we touch, and what touches us also influences our "oral zoo."

These microorganisms communicate with each other using chemical mediators, hormones, and prostaglandins. They share genes with each other and us. They mutate and, by and large, wreak havoc. They are involved in chemical warfare, having the power to modulate their own genes, the genes across species of the organisms they live with, and the genes in you. [Ref 2]

The menagerie in your mouth is so resilient that, after a vigorous teeth cleaning by a dentist, it takes only 24–48 hours for all the bacteria to return—well organized and ready to start creating disease. After home brushing and flossing, it takes only three hours. [Ref 3]

We supply nutrients to the organisms that live in our mouths, and we ingest all of their excrement. Most are parasitic to us or to other organisms we live with. Their toxic effects—and even the bugs themselves—travel in our blood vessels, contributing to strokes, heart attacks, and a plethora of other diseases. [Ref 4 & 5]

But we are getting ahead of ourselves, so let's reflect for a moment on what we have learned:

- Your mouth is teeming with billions of bacteria. Some are good, but many are so caustic or invasive that, under the wrong conditions, they can kill you. They live within a self-defensive, destructive ecosystem on your teeth, gums, and tongue.

- The bacteria that cause periodontal disease are communicable and can be passed from person to person through normal, casual contact.

- To date, the only effective, yet temporary, disruption of this system has been a professional teeth cleaning by a dentist. The cycle of rebuilding the menagerie then begins again within a few hours of leaving the dental chair.

Wouldn't it be great to have a device you could use at home to break this cycle? In Chapters 10 through 13 of this book, you will learn of just such a technology.

Chapter 2

The Biofilm Ecosystem

It's all about biofilm (short for biological film). Biofilm is all around us, particularly in mouths. Bacteria adhere to surfaces in watery environments and then bind themselves to surfaces with their own sticky, glue-like secretion. They consist of many species of organisms—bacteria, fungi, protozoa, and viruses.

Biofilm is a slimy layer teaming with microscopic life. It lives, feeds, grows, excretes, and dies in and on every surface of your teeth, tongue, and mouth. The object of cleaning your teeth is to disrupt this bacterial organization in the mouth before it creates inflammation and disease throughout the rest of your body.

The mouth is a dark, warm, moist environment with a constant temperature and steady supply of nutrients. However, there is only so much space and so many food resources available; therefore, interdependent microorganisms form complex relationships with other species. Fighters and survivors, they seek food and safe shelter and possess an innate desire for procreation.

For optimal health, it is necessary to minimize the biodiversity found in your mouth. Even when teeth are thoroughly cleaned and disinfected, it only takes a few days for the unwanted "guests" described above to completely repopulate through exponential growth. That is why if you don't get your teeth professionally cleaned every three months, you are making a mountain out of a molehill. Small problems in your mouth can quickly spiral into gargantuan issues in your body.

Gaining an upper hand on the biomass in your mouth with a toothbrush and toothpaste is like trying to control an established forest ecosystem with garden clippers. You need powerful tools to get the job done right.

Brushing and flossing do not adequately reduce the biofilm in the areas between teeth and around the gum line, resulting in periodontal disease as the most prevalent disease on the planet. The CDC recently put out the strongest statement in their history that estimates "47.2 percent, or 64.7 million American adults over 30, have mild, moderate, or severe periodontitis." [Ref 6] If you are over 65 years of age, the measurement jumps to 70.1 percent. Periodontal disease has reached epidemic proportions. Later in this book, we will discuss effective solutions to this growing problem.

Chapter 3

Periodontal Disease and Your Body

Periodontal disease comes from the Latin words *peri,* meaning around, and *dontal,* meaning tooth. The bacterial invasion of the tissues around the teeth sets off an inflammatory response from your body while destroying the bone around teeth. This makes them immeasurably more difficult to clean and keep healthy.

Periodontal disease creates an open wound at the tooth and gum interface, providing a portal for organisms to infiltrate your bloodstream and vital organs. The inflammation itself becomes the portal. Blood vessels grow at sites of infection. This is called angiogenesis. The blood vessels transport the bacteria and toxins into your bloodstream, leading to all your organs.

The advance of periodontal disease triggers your body's defense mechanism to inflame your arteries' internal walls by producing cytokines (discussed later). Periodontal problems slowly debilitate the body. The older we get, the worse it gets. People with compromised immune systems need to be extremely vigilant in taking care of their periodontal conditions.

The six signs that can alert one to periodontal disease are:

- Persistent bad breath

- Red or swollen gums

- Tender or bleeding gums

- Painful chewing

- Sensitive teeth

- Loose teeth

Unfortunately, periodontal disease does not show symptoms until it is advanced. Bad breath and bleeding gums are the "canary in the coal mine." You and your dentist, however, can halt its progress.

Periodontal destruction is cumulative. As we age, the infection stresses the heart, lungs, kidneys, pancreas, liver, prostate, and even the brain. Periodontal disease also affects osteoporosis, arthritis, psoriasis, birth weights in infants, and cancers.

Get rid of the infection, and the destruction stops. When we do not see our dentists, as often as recommended, the disease process speeds up and robs us of our longevity. Most periodontal damage becomes increasingly worse the longer dental cleanings are put off, and it is the nature of biofilms to become more disease-provoking as they mature.

Each of us has a unique variation of microbes in our bodies, and genetics also play a role. In a group of people exposed to the same pathogen, some people will succumb to a particular disease, and others will not. Infection or disease occurs when the load of pathogens overwhelms our defense mechanisms, or when the wrong combinations and concentrations of organisms coexist.

The genes of oral bacteria-producing enzymes can alter the function of your own genes producing enzymes. A cascading event occurs when bacteria and viruses in the mouth combine with these entities to alter cell function, tissue function, organ function, and, ultimately, body function. This pathogenic periodontal pathway is much more responsible for life-threatening diseases than we ever realized.

Everything influences our genes. Diet, obesity, environment, exercise—and particularly any infection—switch genes on and off. Since periodontal disease is the most prevalent infection in the majority of all adults, healing this infection pacifies your genes and leads to better overall health.

Higher percentages of shortened lifespans can be attributed to the patch of tissue surrounding your teeth, amounting to nine square inches of gums. Generations of our ancestors have died in ignorance of this chronic infection that can shorten your life and potentially cross-infect your loved ones.

Chapter 4

Periodontal Disease and Your Immune System

Your immune system's job is to produce defensive cells to fight and destroy pathogenic organisms and invading bacteria. Periodontal disease, however, dispatches your immune system into a constant fight with the bacteria from your mouth, forming a state of chronic inflammation.

Cytokines, and especially C-reactive protein (CRP), are the invisible offenders in your body. [Ref 7] CRP indirectly tells your spleen, bone marrow, lymph nodes, adrenal glands, liver, and the blood constituent-making places in your body to produce more of the exact same type of defensive cells that destroy a specific organism or bacteria. The acid and chemical toxins from the excrement of the bacteria bathe the surface layer of teeth and surrounding tissues and trigger your own body's defense mechanism.

This inflammation results in bleeding when your teeth are probed, or sometimes even brushed. One can find these red puffy gums in people from all walks of life.

In short, periodontal disease occurs when these defensive blood cells try to destroy this invasion. It is an excellent response mechanism when you are fighting an acute infection, as we would not survive without this physiological process. With periodontal disease, however, this means your body's immune system is constantly fighting the bugs and, in turn, making your body weak and vulnerable to other systemic diseases. This process taxes the system. Chronic infections that go untreated leave little opportunity for your immune system to combat more acute issues.

Unfortunately, cytokines and CRP caused by advancing periodontal disease also inflame the inner lumen of your blood vessels. This is a major problem if you have a family history of heart disease, or you have compromised circulation in your kidneys, pancreas, or carotids. For diabetic people or those with poor circulation in their legs, this spells real trouble.

Blood flow also transports toxins through the arteries and veins. Therefore, constricted vessels compromise the removal of cellular metabolic waste. When blood is not flushing organs clean of toxins, they are drowning in their own toxins and setting up conditions for malfunction, disease, and even cancer. So chronic elevated CRP negatively affects all the organs in your body.

By now, you recognize that redness around a tooth, sensitivity, odor, loose teeth, and bleeding gums are signs of periodontal disease, a disease that affects your whole body. Bone loss from periodontal disease is generally irreversible without invasive surgery, but can be stopped and controlled with alert and proactive attention to your teeth through regular cleanings and instruction by your dentist or hygienist, and thorough effective biofilm removal.

Chapter 5

Heart Disease and Periodontal Disease

Cardiovascular disease (CVD) claims the life of one American every 37 seconds, according to the American Heart Association's 2009 Heart and Stroke Statistical Update. [Ref 8] CVD includes an assortment of diseases that fall under the general term "heart disease."

Among such diseases are:

- Atherosclerosis (hardening of the arteries caused by calcium deposits and/or fat deposits)

- Heart attack (sudden death of part of the heart)

- Stroke damage to part of the brain (caused by lack of blood oxygen or leakage of blood outside the vessel walls)

- Arrhythmia (abnormal rhythm or rate of heartbeat)

- Angina (heavy, tight squeezing pain in the chest)

- Hypertension (high blood pressure)

- Congestive heart failure (weak heart pumping action causing a buildup of fluid in the lungs and other body tissues)

Rogue genes may lie dormant our entire lives or be expressed under certain conditions. There are risk factors for CVD that one cannot control. These factors include age, gender, and family history. Roughly 80 percent of people who die of heart disease are 65 or older, but it is also the leading cause of death for Americans over the age of 35. Furthermore, those who have a parent with heart disease have a higher risk of developing the disease.

Widely recognized controllable risk factors include smoking, diet, exercise, and alcohol. One lesser-known risk factor is periodontal disease. Atherosclerosis and subsequent CVD are also major concerns for anyone with gum disease. People with periodontitis are twice as likely to die from a heart attack and three times as likely to die from a stroke, according to a study that examined 18 years of medical histories of 1,147 people. [Ref 9]

There are more than 500 research studies and professional reports determining a link between periodontal disease and heart disease. Pamela McClain, DDS, president of the American Academy of Periodontology, sums it up nicely:

Periodontal disease and cardiovascular disease are both complex, multi-factorial diseases that develop over time. It may be overly simplistic to expect a direct causal link. The relationship between the diseases is more likely to be mediated by numerous other factors, mechanisms, and circumstances that we have yet to uncover. [Ref 10]

In addition, Dr. Lauren Patton, professor and chair of the Department of Dental Ecology at the University of North Carolina, wrote, "It is likely the periodontal disease can increase the inflammatory burden, possibly impacting cardiovascular disease... most of the associations with atherosclerosis or atherosclerotic events were modest (10-50% increase in risk)." [Ref 11]

If someone told me that my risk of heart problems could increase by 10 to 50 percent because I also have periodontal disease, I would be on my way to see a dentist pronto.

Furthermore, in February 2013, Dr. Marjorie Jeffcoat conducted a study funded by United Concordia, which showed that heart disease patients who treat their periodontal disease save $2,956 per year in medical expenses. [Ref 12] Clearly, preventing and treating periodontal disease is much less expensive than treating CVD.

Chapter 6

Other Dangers Associated with Periodontal Disease

Stroke

There are about 800,000 stroke victims in the US each year, with more than 140,000 deaths. Strokes are the third leading cause of death, in both men and women, occurring at any age.

Increasing evidence points to the relationship between strokes and periodontal disease. Italian studies have reported that the thickness of the carotid arteries was reduced after treatment for gum disease. The National Center for Biotechnology Information, which published the study, reported that the thickening of the carotid arteries "is positively influenced by periodontal treatment." [Ref 13]

Strokes are most often caused by blockage in a blood vessel, but are also caused by bleeding of a vessel. Studies that acknowledged a link between strokes and periodontal issues showed the strokes were caused by blockages. Calcium and cholesterol deposits in blood vessels break off, cause clotting, and block the blood from reaching the brain. These are often referred to as plaque deposits—not to be confused with periodontal plaque.

Bacteria found in periodontal disease are the perpetrators. While bacteria are in the mouth, the body sets up a defense mechanism to attack the disease. The chemical given off by the body first attacks the periodontal disease, then the proteins in the blood vessels. This irritates and wounds the endothelial cellular lining of all blood vessels. The body's repair, with white blood cells, brings in cholesterol and buildup of arterial plaque in the arteries. When the fatty substances break off from the lining of the blood vessels, they can travel to the brain and block the flow of blood, causing a stroke.

Cancer

Given the importance of inflammation in the creation of tumors and angiogenesis (creation of blood vessels, which is a problem in cancers), more studies need to be performed. According to an article written by Karen S. Sfanos, MD (Department of Pathology, Sidney Kimmel Comprehensive Cancer Center, the Johns Hopkins University School of Medicine), and Angelo M. De Marzo, MD (Adjunct Professor of Pathology and Oncology, the Johns Hopkins University School of Medicine):

Chronic inflammation is now known to contribute to several forms of human cancer, with an estimated 20% of adult cancers attributable to chronic inflammatory conditions caused by infectious agents, chronic non-infectious inflammatory diseases and/or other environmental factors. Indeed, chronic inflammation is now regarded as an "enabling characteristic" of human cancer. [Ref 14]

Do not wait for the data to point to the cause of your personal systemic affliction. Treat the systemic inflammation that is occurring below your gum line and in between your teeth now.

Research published in the Journal of Molecular Cell Biology found that a long-term lack of oxygen in cells may be a key driver of cancer growth. [Ref 15]

Cancer growth is caused by the direct effect that long-term CRP production has on the cells lining the internal vessel walls (endothelium lining), causing constriction of the vessel due to inflammation. Constriction lowers blood flow to all vital organs—CRP is primarily responsible—and a clot forms. Sometimes it causes a blockage at the site, and sometimes it breaks away and flows to another area of your body. An embolus chokes the blood supply, starving tissue of oxygen.

Peripheral Arterial Disease (PAD)

Although many studies have been conducted on the relationship between periodontal disease and heart disease, in general, few studies have been done on Peripheral Arterial Disease (PAD) and its relation to periodontal disease.

The Mayo Clinic defines PAD as:

A common circulatory problem in which narrowed arteries reduce blood flow to your limbs. Extremities—usually your legs—do not receive enough blood flow to keep up with demand. This causes symptoms, most notably leg pain when walking.

Peripheral artery disease is also likely to be a sign of a more widespread accumulation of fatty deposits in your arteries (atherosclerosis). This condition may be reducing blood flow to your heart and brain, as well as your legs.

A 2012 study reported in the Journal of Periodontology found that subjects with periodontal disease were six times more likely to have PAD than subjects without periodontal disease. This supports an earlier 1980/1990 study that concluded men with periodontal disease had a significantly higher risk of PAD. [Ref 16]

Diabetes

Evidence supports that the relationship between diabetes and periodontal diseases is bidirectional. That is to say, poor control over blood sugar has a negative impact on periodontal disease, and periodontal disease has a negative impact on blood sugar control in diabetic patients. [Ref 17]

Diabetes affects about 25 million Americans, and another 7 million are undiagnosed. It is characterized by high levels of blood sugar caused by malfunctioning insulin production. An insulin-resistant individual becomes diabetic when the pancreas can no longer put out a sufficient amount of insulin to lower the blood sugar, and the organ becomes exhausted. [Ref 18]

The pancreas is controlled by hormonal feedback mechanisms. Acute and chronic infections create hormonal chaos in the body. Blood vessels in a diabetic are also compromised. They thicken and slow the delivery of oxygen to the extremities, likewise slowing the removal of waste from these tissues. These actions lower the defense response to infection, including periodontal infection.

Both adults and children with diabetes have more severe periodontal issues, and those with periodontal disease have a more difficult time controlling their diabetes. About 50 percent of all children have some form of periodontal disease, according to the Lucile Packard Children's Hospital at Stanford University Medical Center. [Ref 19] It is especially important that those with diabetes receive regular oral check-ups and be treated for periodontal infection.

A study at the School of Dental Medicine at the University of Buffalo found that obesity is significantly related to periodontal disease through the pathway of insulin resistance. Sara Grossi, director of the UB Periodontal Disease Research Center and lead author of the study, said, "Now we see a relationship between obesity, insulin resistance and periodontal disease in a large, population-based cohort. This relationship is significant because obesity is an important risk factor for Type 2 diabetes and heart disease." [Ref 20]

Diabetics can also save money by practicing thorough oral hygiene. A study by Cigna Insurance showed that periodontal treatment given to people with diabetes saved more than $2,400 per year, or 23 percent, in their healthcare costs. [Ref 21]

United Concordia, a dental insurance carrier, and High-mark, a medical insurance carrier, examined claims from 1.7 million patients and found that those with diabetes who treated their periodontal disease spent an average of $1,477 per year less on prescription drugs, and $1,814 per year less on hospital and doctor visits, compared to those diabetics who did not see a dentist. [Ref 22]

Today, adults and children with diabetes have a good chance of keeping this disease under control. Besides a proper diet, diligence and thoroughness in oral health is also necessary. More studies on this relationship are needed to ascertain the effect these conditions have on one another.

COPD

Chronic Obstructive Pulmonary Disease (COPD) is a general term referring to inflammatory lung disease. The air sacs of the lung lose elasticity and the bronchioles pro-duce thick mucus, which creates a chronic cough. Airflow is restricted and lung congestion occurs due to this excessive mucus production. Shortness of breath is frequent. COPD limits normal everyday functions. Periodontal pathogens can exacerbate the disease by infiltrating the bronchioles through aspiration into the upper pharyngeal region or airway, causing pneumonia in compromised patients. As in periodontal disease, the overreaction of the inflammatory process occurs and the lung's connective tissue further breaks down, preventing a healthy exchange of oxygen.

Some 16 million Americans suffer from COPD, the sixth leading cause of death in the United States. F. Scannapieco, DMD, lead researcher of a study published in January 2001 in the Journal of Periodontology, found that patients with periodontal disease have a 1.5 times greater risk of COPD. [Ref 23]

As we age, our lung capacity decreases and oral bacteria compromise the exchange of oxygen with carbon dioxide. The common theme here is inflammation. [Ref 24]

Pregnancy

Women with periodontal disease have a 7.5 times higher risk of delivering a premature baby of low birth weight. [Ref 25] Studies have also shown that poor oral health can delay fertility by two months. [Ref 26] An extensive and ongoing United Concordia study on healthcare costs found a 73.7 percent decrease, or $2,433 cost savings, for women who were pregnant and treated their gum disease. [Ref 27] Finally, pregnant women need to be inflammatory disease free, since oral microbes cross the placental barrier.

Breast Cancer

New data concerning women's health has linked periodontal disease to breast cancer. This came from an extensive, long-term study concluded in October 2010 in Huddinge, Sweden, by the Karolinska Institute's Department of Dental Medicine, Division of Periodontology. More than 3,000 women between the ages of 30 and 40 years old were part of a 16-year randomized study. "Of the subjects with periodontal disease with any missing molars in the mandible, 5.5% had breast cancer, in comparison to 0.5% of the subjects who had periodontal disease but no missing molars," the study reported. Missing molars are a sign of long-term periodontal issues. [Ref 28]

One explanation is that the bacteria from periodontal disease infect the entire blood supply of patients with advanced periodontal disease. This infection then sets off viral infections, referred to as "co-infections." These other infections cause the body to use its entire immune response to fight the co-infections, leaving a suppressed immune system to fight off the cancer. This information will not surprise those in the medical field who have long known that periodontal disease affects the whole body.

Arthritis

Several studies examining the relationship between rheumatoid arthritis and periodontal disease have been conducted in the past 10 years. Perhaps the strongest statement made by any of the studies was from Australia, reported in the Journal of Periodontology: "The results of this study provide further evidence of a significant association between periodontitis and rheumatoid arthritis." [Ref 29]

Again, in the United Concordia study of healthcare costs related to periodontal disease, Dr. Jeffcoat found that annual medical costs were $3,964 lower for rheumatoid arthritis patients who treated their periodontal disease. [Ref 30]

As with periodontal disease and other systemic diseases, rheumatoid arthritis is an inflammatory disease. One inflammatory disease that produces high levels of CRP exacerbates the other. This is also true of arthritis.

Alzheimer's

Spirochetes have been found in the brains of Alzheimer's patients, according to a study published in the Journal of Neuroinflammation. [Ref 31] Other viruses and bacteria, as well as the toxins from the spirochetes, are suspected to be co-contributors to the chronic inflammation. In the study, the onset of the spirochete infection occurred long before a diagnosis of dementia or Alzheimer's. Other studies confirm that inflammation is a prevalent feature in the brains of Alzheimer's victims. Proteins from the virus initiate inflammation. Viruses are responsible for immune activation in many diseases, including Alzheimer's.

Both periodontal disease and Alzheimer's disease are multifactorial infections likely influenced by a multitude of variables.

We see periodontal disease and its inherent dangers associated with a long list of deadly health problems, and many of these health issues affect both children and adults. This is not science fiction. Your mouth and what is growing, living, and dying in it is a constant delivery system to your organs, major systems, and entire body. Traditional home dental care simply does not do enough to control the zoo in your mouth and reduce the impact of periodontal disease on your body.

Go to www.dentalairforce.com to read extensive articles on the relationship between periodontal disease and other diseases.

Chapter 7

Put Your Money Where Your Mouth Is

The mouth is important in every aspect of your life. It is the first line of communication to your vital organs, and because periodontal disease is contagious, your mouth can influence the health of your entire family.

Caring for patients for more than 30 years has given me a special lens through which I view the world. Thorough dental cleanings four times a year are probably the best things you can do for your mouth. Even as far back as 1978, dental researchers realized that twice-a-year cleanings are not adequate.

Many people do not want to pay for dental work necessary for long-term solutions to their health problems. It is not too late to put your money where your mouth is and reap valuable dividends for the rest of your life.

Here's another way of looking at this concept: The treatment of inflammation and the complications from periodontal disease are two huge moneymakers for pharmaceutical companies. While it is easy to throw drugs at inflammation, it is more effective and less expensive to deal with the source of the problem—the biofilm. Let's look at what we spend on just one class of pharmaceutical drugs compared to what is spent on all of dentistry.

The US Centers for Disease Control and Prevention reports that about 16 percent of US adults use statins.

Statin drugs are cholesterol-lowering medications, such as Lipitor®, Pravachol®, and Crestor®. Statins are one of the most controversial therapies in the medical industry. Why? Many studies show statin drugs do not significantly lower your risk of a heart attack. Indeed, statins may exacerbate many other problems and can result in death. Years ago, cholesterol was said to be the main culprit of heart disease. Pharmaceutical companies were quick to deliver this message. Since making a drug to lower cholesterol is as easy as blocking a liver enzyme, statins have become the largest revenue-producing and most profitable drug in history. Some statins have a 500,000 percent profit margin! An estimated 34 million people in the US spend more than $30 billion in a year on statins.

And this is only one type of drug! Yet, this is one third of what is spent on the entire dental market, including appointments, radiographs, cleanings, fillings, root canals, crowns, periodontal therapy, and implants. Is the culprit cholesterol, which is present in every cell in your body, or is it inflammation?

As we age, plaque builds up in our arteries. For many decades, cardiologists cited saturated fats and cholesterol as the cause of plaque deposits, and indeed, they are half right. Now cardiologists characterize this vascular disease as a general inflammatory process. Diet and lack of exercise exacerbate this natural condition of aging.

Fortunately, cardiologists now look at CRP levels more than high cholesterol levels and refer their patients to dentists, who can reduce chronic inflammation and lower CRP levels, or look for other areas of infection. It is also interesting to note that periodontal disease shifts from mild to moderate around the age of 40, which is the same age when medical doctors begin to treat rising blood cholesterol levels and prescribe statins.

The key to lowering coronary artery disease is lowering CRP and cytokine levels. Inflammation, combined with cholesterol, causes the heart attacks. Where is this bodily inflammation coming from? The Centers for Disease Control says that 50 percent of the population over 30 years of age has periodontal disease, so there is likely a strong correlation between CRP levels and periodontal disease.

Considering the amount of toxins entering your body from periodontal disease, a better way to reduce inflammation is by eliminating the cause—not masking the symptoms with drugs.

Simply put: controlling periodontal disease is the easiest and least expensive way to modify your risk factors for many potentially deadly diseases. Using Dental Air Force can improve the general health of your mouth, reduce the germs that create periodontal disease, and improve your overall health.

Chapter 8

Healthcare—Dental Care

Healthcare has traditionally been essentially blind to dental care. Most healthcare programs discuss how costs should be contained or lowered by focusing on treatments. This includes lowering Medicaid and Medicare reimbursements, paying doctors based on their performance in hospitals, and purchasing innovative medical devices (robotics) to provide more predictable outcomes and treat patients more quickly and efficiently.

In the past, very little was mentioned about prevention when discussing lowering healthcare costs. It seemed that medical and insurance communities were stuck in one lane of traffic, chasing chronic diseases. The tolls along that road keep getting more and more expensive. Once a person has diseases associated with chronic inflammation (or high CRP), such as heart disease, diabetes, and lung disease, treatment typically continues for decades. However, to lower the burden on the system, prevention can replace costly treatment.

When will people realize that great oral care is a bargain that provides health and longevity? How can anything that is right under our noses escape the rationale of wisdom-seekers, the prowess of number-crunching accountants, the notice of healers, and the work of physicians and dentists?

Just one example of cost savings in the total healthcare picture is treating periodontal disease in diabetics. In the previously mentioned United Concordia study, patients with diabetes who treated their periodontal disease saved almost $2,840 per year in total medical costs compared to those who did not. [Ref 32]

It is time to cover periodontal therapy through healthcare insurance instead of dental insurance. It makes sense for both patients and insurance companies because of the indisputable link between periodontal disease and other systemic diseases of the major organs.

Oral disease is anything but localized. A study in Japan showed that overall healthcare costs were 21 percent higher for subjects with periodontal disease. [Ref 33] How many dollars, not to mention lives, could be saved through proper care? According to the Center for Medicare & Medicaid Services, in 2010, individuals, corporations, and the United States local, state, and federal governments spent $2.6 trillion on healthcare. [Ref 34]

That is $8,402 per year for every man, woman, and child. This amount represents 17.9 percent of our Gross Domestic Product. The healthcare savings according to the Japanese study are 21 percent. Multiply 21 percent by $2.6 trillion and it equals $546 billion.

Since the US government pays 28 percent of that $2.6 trillion healthcare bill, it alone would reap 28 percent of the $546 billion dollar savings, or $153 billion, if health insurance companies covered periodontal therapy. In addition, there would be an increase in productivity of the healthy individuals who pay taxes.

Many people do not want to pay for the work that is necessary for healthy long-term solutions to their issues, but cardiologists, diabetic physicians, or other medical professionals may require you to have your periodontal disease treated. The cost of periodontal treatment varies between $1,200 to $2,500 for a two-year treatment plan. It should make you angry that your health insurance does not cover it. After all, these companies cover all sorts of other life-threatening, systemic diseases. Since, according to medical textbooks, your mouth is part of your gastrointestinal system, how did oral care get dropped from overall healthcare coverage?

United Concordia is one medical healthcare insurance company that understands the consequences of periodontal disease to their policyholders. In July 2013, they introduced policies that provide 100 percent coverage of periodontal therapy. They are truly pioneers in recognizing the whole body connection and doing what is right for their clients.

It is time other insurance companies follow United Concordia's example. We should all push insurance companies and bureaucratic healthcare companies to look at the research linking periodontal disease to many deadly diseases and to start treating the body as one complete system.

Cleaning your teeth with Dental Air Force provides a higher quality of life. I like to say it buys you birthdays.

Chapter 9

Toothbrushes, Toothpaste, and Cleaning Habits

Teeth are like loved ones. When your teeth are gone, you are going to miss them. Today, you have a very good chance to live to be 100 years old, so ask yourself:

- How have I done so far?
- Have my teeth been cared for enough in my past to get me to the end of the line?
- Have I neglected my dental condition and, unwittingly, shortened my life because of it?

Having teeth when you are 70 or older will make your life more joyful. Think about what your teeth will be like in ten years. What would you give for the teeth you had when you were 20, or before your first cavity? Have you given your teeth the necessary care to get you to 100?

The major reason teeth don't last is because we do not do a very good job cleaning them. In fact, out of 100 people brushing their teeth, every one of them will achieve a different level of cleanliness. This is mostly because people have different brushing habits. Some will miss the same spots repeatedly and over-abrade other spots. The cheek surface of the back teeth is a prime example. We brush so hard that we damage the root surface. Then we use our tongue as a gauge for "cleanliness," but our tongues are huge and, like the toothbrush, do not have access to sites between our teeth.

Here are some variables:

- the brush
- the toothpaste
- the pressure used
- the technique, the frequency, and the time spent
- how often you receive professional cleanings

Other variables include the basic structure of your teeth, their condition, and your age. Are you consistent with your daily home cleanings? What is your diet like? Do you have the full gambit of dental work—crowns, fillings between teeth, root canals, a partial, a bridge, implants, braces, or periodontal disease?

There is a science to cleaning teeth. You can control the outcome with proper time, frequency, and thoroughness. All of the variables make the job of cleaning teeth more difficult than you may have thought.

Most people are doing as much damage as good with their toothbrush and toothpaste, leaving roughly 40 percent of each tooth untouched. This means they are at best 60 percent clean—actually, they are super-clean in a small area, abused and over-abraded.

There is also the biofilm contamination issue with a toothbrush. The bristles of a brush are teeming with bacteria from the last time you used it. "The area of the toothbrush in which tufts are anchored is especially prone to contamination," says Dr. Rajiv Saini, periodontist, PHD researcher, and Editor in Chief, IJEDS. Contaminated toothbrushes inoculate healthy sites. Biofilm grows and burrows into your soft tissue, hard tissue, and bloodstream day after day after day.

Most of my patients 40 years or older have inflammation and damage to the sides of their teeth due to over-abrasion. This often results in a groove at the junction of the teeth and gums. One study on the prevalence of non-carious cervical lesions showed that 53 percent of the participants were affected by the ravages of the toothbrush. [Ref 35]

As you age, the statistics get worse—in older groups, up to 85 percent have this abrasion. Toothbrush abrasion causes the sharp pain you feel when eating something cold, hot, acidic, or sweet, because the surface is devoid of protective enamel. Since the nerve lies closer to the root surface than it does to the enamel, it becomes painful. Overzealous tooth brushing is usually the culprit.

The inadequate brushing habits we acquire as kids seem to be okay until we are 30 or 40 years old. Then, all of a sudden, patients come in and say, "This tooth is sensitive," thinking it is something that has just occurred when, in reality, the damage has been in the making for 25 years.

That is why studies show that brushing teeth for four minutes gets them no cleaner than if you brush them for two minutes. You are simply over-abrading the already clean surfaces and never reaching the most critical surfaces of the tooth. The biofilm left in these areas re-contaminates clean areas immediately.

Toothpastes seem to be the culprit as much as the brush itself, especially if you ask the toothbrush manufactures.

Since the 1970s, toothpastes have become more and more abrasive. However, if you ask toothpaste companies what causes abrasion, they will tell you it is the brush. Nobody is sued (although it has been tried) and it doesn't really matter. Both industries will argue it was your technique that caused the problem. It is really a multifactorial issue—brush, paste, technique, and repetition ruin your teeth.

The bristles of a brush drag toothpaste granules across the teeth, resulting in scratches on the dentin and surface of the enamel. Gouges in tooth dentin leave teeth vulnerable to acid erosion. One of the reasons teeth become sensitive is that microbes on your teeth secrete acid, lower the pH at that site, and begin to erode the enamel in these grooves. Drinks or foods that have a pH below 5.5—orange juice, candy, and even some bottled drinking waters—can also cause this sensitivity.

As humans, we are very adaptable and can get used to almost anything. We learn to guard our exposed roots with our cheeks or tongues when we drink cold or hot beverages.

Some toothpaste products market themselves solely using anti-sensitivity propaganda. In reality, these desensitizing toothpastes mask the underlying issues, further perpetuating dental destruction. The symptom is alleviated—the area does not feel sensitive—but the groove becomes bigger and creeps closer to the nerve.

Some of the sensitivity may also develop because of the sodium lauryl sulfate found in almost all toothpastes. This chemical is a foaming agent and is very irritating to the groove and soft tissue. It is responsible for many soft tissue ulcers and chronic mild rashes that are intraoral or around the lips.

As far as root surfaces are concerned, the only thing you will get "fresh" out of your toothpaste is a layer of exposed dental tubules. After the root is exposed due to toothbrush abrasion, chemical erosion occurs after eating acidic foods or drinks, which etch exposed dentin on the surface of the root. Organic components of the exposed root are washed away, leaving frail crystals or shards pointing up on the surface like a carpet of fragile stalagmites. Then the toothpaste and toothbrush combination plows through and knocks off any points left behind. This repetitive destruction and demineralization forms a groove in the side of the tooth at the gum line. This spells "ouch" to hot and cold and sweets, and bacterial invasion.

If you are using an electric toothbrush, you are just speeding up the damage. A brush is a brush. Putting power to it—whether it is spinning, pulsing, or vibrating—is not going to change the fundamental flaw in toothbrushes. If toothbrushes are not doing the job, it is imperative to find a solution.

Chapter 10

The Development of Dental Air Force

History of Hygiene

Here is a very short history of the advancements for personal dental hygiene over the centuries.

3500 BC—Twigs from aromatic trees and other natural materials are used to clean teeth.

2700 BC—The Chinese start using forms of mouthwash, with agents like saltwater and vinegar, to clean teeth.

1780—The first toothbrush is created in England from swine bone and hog bristles.

1852—US dentist Levi Parmly creates dental floss for getting debris out from between teeth.

1873—Colgate introduces mass-produced toothpaste in a bottle, then, in 1890, introduces toothpaste in a tube.

1914—Toothpaste fluoride is introduced to help prevent decay.

1939—The modern nylon bristle toothbrush is introduced.

1954—The electric toothbrush is invented.

1962—Waterpik hits the market to flush out food particles from between teeth.

That is about it. We have had nine notable advances in personal oral hygiene over 5,500 years. No wonder the average American spends less than four minutes a day taking care of his or her teeth.

You now have a better understanding of the hundreds of billions of bacteria in your mouth that you have to keep at bay daily with so few tools. You also have an idea why we need a better way to take care of our teeth. To the nine advancements in personal dental care, we now add Dental Air Force—a major leap forward in managing oral hygiene.

The advantage of Dental Air Force over a toothbrush is that it uses a targeted jet of air, water, and dental cleaner to access the tiniest spaces between teeth and along the gum lines. As discussed, all toothbrushes miss a lot of those spots, and brushing also tends to be over aggressive on some surfaces of teeth (the cheek side) while being under aggressive on other areas.

Dental Air Force eliminates the issue of over-abrading and easily accesses the difficult-to-reach areas. Another big difference between Dental Air Force and a toothbrush is that your brush bristles harbor bacteria for chronic inoculation every time you use it.

In fact, clinical studies showed that Dental Air Force removes 62 percent more plaque-producing bacteria between teeth than the leading power toothbrush. (Unpublished, available on www.dentalairforce.com)

Achieving a New Level of Oral Health

It has taken my entire professional career to actualize Dental Air Force. The epiphany that inspired the idea for Dental Air Force came early in my career.

All dentists practice differently, based on where they went to school, when they were educated, and who mentored them. I started out focusing on restorative work. My forte was crown and bridge and posterior gold work. With time and continued education, I gravitated toward prevention and periodontal disease therapy.

Originally, I had a hygienist and two assistants, and I provided the staff with the best equipment possible to make their jobs efficient. A couple of years into the practice, I bought a device called a Prophy-Jet® for my hygienist to clean teeth and remove stains. But like many instruments and supplies, the device went unused for a number of reasons.

Once while my hygienist was on leave, I jumped in and started doing hygiene cleanings myself—something most dentists feel is below their station. I tried the Prophy-Jet® and could not believe how well it worked—the stains disappeared like magic! In fact, it worked so well that one day I thought, everybody should have one of these in their home for everyday use. It would eliminate the very difficult-to-repair toothbrush abrasion evident in almost every mouth, and effectively clean in between teeth.

Developing Dental Air Force and getting FDA clearance for marketing was a monumental task that I became mentally, physically, and financially immersed in for two decades. I am proud to say it is the first and only medical device to receive FDA clearance for marketing as a replacement for tooth brushing and oral irrigators.

By coming up with a more impactful solution to this world-wide problem of preventing periodontal disease, I feel I have served my profession well and reached beyond my small family of patients to have a profound impact on the overall health of a much greater population. Anyone who buys Dental Air Force is my patient.

Dental Air Force now provides everyone, with or without dental insurance, the opportunity to achieve a new level of hygiene for themselves and their families. Using Dental Air Force is your dental insurance.

That is how and why I created Dental Air Force. It is a home dental cleaning appliance that provides a completely new way to clean your teeth between professional cleanings.

Visit www.dentalairforce.com for more information.

Chapter 11

Using Dental Air Force

Dental Air Force consists of a base about the size of a toaster. This base houses a compressor that provides the air source delivered through the hand piece. Air mixes with the dental cleaner and delivers it at high speed through the hand piece tip to power wash the teeth, between teeth, the gum lines, and hard-to-reach places in your mouth.

Simple to Set Up, Easy to Use

The key parts of Dental Air Force can be set up and ready to use right out of the box in less than 10 minutes.

To use Dental Air Force, you simply place dental cleaner in the hand piece bottle, add water or hydrogen peroxide, shake, and you are ready to start. Your teeth will be cleaner the first time you use Dental Air Force, because the device immediately removes more biofilm, plaque, and debris between teeth than a toothbrush and toothpaste ever will.

Dental Air Force Versus Oral Irrigators and Flossing

Dental Air Force is very different from a Waterpik or any oral irrigator. Oral irrigators use only water to try to remove plaque. Plaque, however, is very much like grease and resists removal with just water. The FDA-cleared for marketing Dental Air Force uses air, dental cleaner, and a water jet to break through plaque barriers. Air oxygenates the spaces between teeth and along the gum line, making it difficult for the anaerobic, plaque-causing bacteria to live. Sodium bicarbonate in the cleaner is a neutralizing agent that acts on the acids produced by the bacteria. It also acts as an abrasive, breaking up the plaque's sticky film and removing the odor caused by the plaque. Water flushes bacteria and debris off teeth surfaces. Oral irrigators were developed to remove food debris from between teeth. Dental Air Force replaces tooth brushing and oral irrigators.

American Dental Association (ADA) surveys reveal that less than 5 percent of people floss. And research shows only 18-35 percent of plaque is actually removed by flossing. So basically, floss isn't working, either. Dental Air Force combines both tooth brushing and oral irrigating in one procedure.

Dental Air Force Cleaner

Home care is even more important than professional cleanings because it occurs daily. Dental Air Force is designed to modify the biofilm environment between teeth—where the most complex and virulent biofilm resides—by oxygenating around the teeth and down into periodontal pockets.

All the ingredients in the Dental Air Force cleaner are natural. The dental cleaner is a powder that contains sodium bicarbonate, natural mint flavoring, xylitol, stevia, guar and xanthan gums, and calcium triphosphate. Sodium bicarbonate is baking soda. Xylitol is a sweetener that also has anti-cavity properties, stevia is a natural non-caries sweetener, the gums suspend the particles for even application, and calcium triphosphate remineralizes enamel.

Sodium bicarbonate alters the environment by raising the pH in between the teeth, inhibiting the growth of anaerobic bacteria. The jet stream of air increases the oxygen concentration at the sites between the teeth and below the gum line. The system also uses air with sodium bicarbonate particles to disrupt biofilm cells and reduce their tenacity. This results in remineralization, along with healthier enamel and root surfaces.

Whitens Your Teeth as You Clean

When you replace the water in the dental cleaner cup with over-the-counter hydrogen peroxide and clean your teeth twice a day, you can, over a one-month period, achieve the same results as professional whitening. The whitening effect accumulates over time and is the preferred method for bleaching teeth, since hydrogen peroxide will not shock the teeth as does a one-time bleaching process. Additional benefits are the continuous and routine disinfection and oxidation of teeth and tissue.

Works Great With Braces, Crowns, Bridges, and Implants

Dental Air Force is particularly effective on orthodontic appliances and crowns, bridges, and implants. These restorations and hardware make your teeth even harder to clean with a brush. Imagine the difference between power washing your porch deck versus using a broom. Which is going to do a superior job? If you were using a broom on your deck, you would scratch through the wood before you could clean between the boards. Dental Air Force gets into all the tiny cracks and crevices where a toothbrush just cannot reach, without damaging the enamel or cutting into the root surfaces.

Dental Air Force is a remarkably effective tool as an adjunct in the treatment of periodontal disease. It will not cure the disease, nor substitute for professional treatment of the disease. No one device or procedure is going to provide the miracle cure. Dental Air Force does, however, augment the professional dentist treatment of periodontal disease and is one of the best tools you can use at home.

To receive our articles on periodontal disease, register at www.dentalairforce.com.

People who use Dental Air Force are absolutely convinced they have found the best way to keep their teeth clean and white and their gums healthy between visits to the dentist. Here are some testimonials about their experiences with the total cleaning power of Dental Air Force:

"Dental Air Force inhibits the cause of many systemic diseases in an elegant and thorough fashion and is a life saver. By the regular use of Dental Air Force home dental cleaning system, there will be improvement in the systemic health of the individual users and the diseases that are associated with periodontal diseases will be controlled or prevented for longer duration of time."

-Rajiv Saini, periodontist—Maharashtra, India

"You've made me a believer! Prior to using Dental Air Force, I consistently brushed, flossed, and followed doctors' orders, but still had two gum surgeries for periodontal disease. However, since using DAF for six years, my hygienist says I always have very healthy gums. Also, my teeth used to be very sensitive (even when using special toothpaste). Now I have no sensitivity issues."

-Jerry—Dahlonega, GA

"Normally, I will not take the time to write a company about a product, however, the Dental Air Force is worth the accolades. My dentist and orthodontist encouraged me to purchase the Dental Air Force for two reasons: receding gums due to excessive brushing, and cleaning my braces. Your amazing product completely removed stains and left my acrylic braces as white as snow! My only regret is that we waited and didn't buy it sooner."

-Susan—Holland, MI

"Thank you for your excellent service and an amazing product. My twice-yearly cleanings are a breeze, and my dentist always comments on my excellent oral health. Anyone who values his or her dental health should use a DAF!"

-Dawn—Anchorage, AK

"The Dental Air Force is great. It is like visiting the dentist and receiving a professional cleaning daily. Thanks for a great product."

-Henry—Ayer, MA

Chapter 12

Dental Air Force Studies

Dental Air Force consistently yielded remarkable results when it underwent the following published and unpublished studies for Food and Drug Administration (FDA) clearance for marketing:

1. Testing its effectiveness in removing bacteria-causing plaque from all tooth surfaces: The power toothbrush/toothpaste combination was very aggressive in removing bacteria-causing plaque on the easily accessed cheek side and tongue side tooth surfaces, but failed to remove bacteria-causing plaque in between teeth. Dental Air Force equally removed bacteria-causing plaque from all three surfaces of teeth, and was especially effective in eliminating bacteria-causing plaque between teeth. (Unpublished, available on www.dentalairforce.com).

2. Safety when used on soft tissue (gums): The abrasion was markedly less with Dental Air Force than from either the powered or manual toothbrush cleanings. (Unpublished, available on www.dentalairforce.com).

3. Abrasiveness on tooth dentin: Dental Air Force tested safe on tooth dentin and root surfaces. (Unpublished, available on www.dentalairforce.com).

4. CRP levels or blood markers for inflammation study: After using a toothbrush and paste following periodontal therapy, CRP levels remained the same after three months. However, when using Dental Air Force after the periodontal treatment, CRP levels continued to drop throughout the six-month study. [Ref 36]

5. Diabetic study testing for glycated hemoglobin (A1c): Dental Air Force, as an adjunct to periodontal therapy, achieved a significantly improved reduction in glycated hemoglobin than the toothbrush. [Ref 37]

A major United Kingdom Prospective Diabetes Study, published in 2000, quantified many of the benefits of reducing a high HbA1c level by as little as 1 percent. They reported: [Ref 38]

- A 16% decrease in risk of heart failure
- A 14% decrease in risk of fatal or nonfatal heart attack
- A 12% decrease in risk of fatal or nonfatal stroke
- A 21% decrease in risk of diabetes-related death
- A 14% decrease in risk of death from all causes
- A 43% decrease in risk of amputation

- A 37% decrease in risk of small blood vessel disease

Conclusion: Using Dental Air Force can help decrease your A1c levels by more than 1 percent and save your life, or certainly extend it.

6. Microbial study testing the load of pathogens below the gum line: After six months, the Dental Air Force group had one fifth of the periodontal pathogens than the toothbrush group. [Ref 39]

7. Basic clinical parameters such as bleeding and gum attachment levels study: Each parameter measured showed that after Phase 1 periodontal therapy, Dental Air Force performed better than the toothbrush. [Ref 40]

Every one of these seven studies showed Dental Air Force positively influencing local and systemic health. For details of specific studies, please email your request to office@dentalairforce.com.

Chapter 13

Conclusion

The simple truth? Preventing advancing periodontal disease will help you live longer and give you a better quality of life.

As we age, we begin to see there is not much gold in those golden years. Injuries take more and more time to heal. Our hair gets thinner and thinner. Our memories get shorter and shorter. Our reflexes slow down. We age fast enough without having a chronic inflammatory disease to speed things up.

Historically, each time societies have increased cleanliness or hygiene, we have increased our longevity. We are living longer, but with more diseases.

Heart disease and cancer are the culprits that shorten our lives. We are just discovering how viruses interact with the bugs or bacteria in your mouth and cripple your defense mechanism to fight cancer and heart disease. Pick up any book on the Middle Ages and read about the disgusting living conditions and lack of hygiene. The life expectancy then was the same as when Christ was on earth—30 years. During the twentieth century, we went from a life expectancy of 50 years to 77.5 years. This was due to our awareness and development of hygiene practices, use of vaccinations, and the discovery of a bug-killing, life-saving, world-changing, and interventional medicine called "penicillin."

The mouth is the last frontier for hygiene. Increasing hygiene in this area will provide the next leap in our longevity. It is only been during the last 20 years that we have recognized that oral hygiene impacts the entire body. Oral hygiene affects the cardiovascular system and every organ in the body. It is an inflammatory, systemic disease that is contagious, infectious, and communicable. This knowledge should awaken us to the fact that our oral hygiene requires more than what a toothbrush, floss, and the six-month professional cleanings provide. It is a lingering 1950's mentality that keeps us in a pattern of six-month cleanings. If you want to increase your life span, see your dentist every three months.

There is amazing return on investment (ROI) when you put your money where your mouth is. You live longer, and that is big time at the end of the line. You live healthier the whole way through if you get into an oral fitness program now.

Prevention is the key to unlocking the vault of longevity within each of us.

Data in Studies

Studies exploring inflammation present in periodontal disease and its link with a multitude of other systemic diseases are piling up. Are you going to wait until the evidence has been tested for 50 years to do something about it? Who knows how long it will be before researchers unequivocally and indisputably claim that periodontal disease is indeed a root cause of certain specific cancers and other systemic diseases. Not 80 percent of the population smokes. Not 80 percent of the population drinks. Not 80 percent of the population is genetically pre-disposed to specific cancers. BUT 80 percent of the population has some form of gum disease. Given these interactions with other factors and the growing research showing a connection between periodontal disease and many life-threatening diseases, why would you not do everything that is available to prevent and treat inflammation in the mouth, or periodontal disease?

As new discoveries are made, do not expect the medical community to jump on the bandwagon. Studies involving smoking and cancer are a great example of the government and medical field dragging their feet. How many quantifiable research studies needed to be done before the general public was made aware that smoking causes cancer? In 1912, it was suggested that lung cancer was caused from smoking. And by 1929, quantitative studies were rolling in, yet it was not until 1964 that the Surgeon General concluded that smoking is a cause of lung disease.

So we have years to go before the medical field will act on all the data showing the associations of periodontal disease and systemic diseases and promote the public to throw away their toothbrushes. It will likely take Dental Air Force decades to replace the toothbrush. Progress works at a snail's pace. Writing this book will be a catalyst to further disseminate change. Please share this information with friends and family members.

REFERENCES

1 Mahanonda, Rangsini, Noppadol Sa-Ard-Iam, Pimprapa Rerkyen, Chantrakorn Champaiboon, and Narisara Vanavit. "Innate antiviral immunity of periodontal tissue." Periodontology 2000 56.1 (2011): 143–53. Web. 18 June 2013.

2 Saini, Rajiv, Santosh Saini, and Sugandha Sharma. "Biofilm: A dental microbial infection." Journal of Natural Science, Biology and Medicine 2.1 (2011): 71–75. Web. 16 May 2013.

3 Addy, Martin, and Patrick Adriaens. "Epidemiology and Etiology of Periodontal Diseases and the Role of Plaque Control in Dental Caries." Proceedings of the European Workshop on Mechanical Plaque Control. Ed. Niklaus P. Lang, Rolf Attström, and Harald Löe. First ed. Chicago: Quintessence Publishing, 1998. 98–101. Print.

4 Ohki, Takahiro, Yuji Itabashi, Takashi Kohno, Akihiro Yoshizawa, and Shuichi Nishikubo. "Detection of periodontal bacteria in thrombi of patients with acute myocardial infarction by polymerase chain reaction." American Heart Journal 163.2 (2012): 164–67. Web. 18 June 2013.

5 Haynes, William G., and Clark Stanford. "Periodontal Disease and Atherosclerosis: From Dental to Arterial Plaque." Editorial. Arteriosclerosis, Thrombosis, and Vascular Biology 23.8 (2003): 1309–11. Web. 18 June 2013.

6 "CDC: Half of American Adults Have Periodontal Disease." Perio.org. Ed. Kenneth S. Kornman. American Academy of Periodontology, 4 September 2012. Web. 16 May 2013.

7 "Inflammation: Chronic." Life Extension. Life Extension, 2013. Web. 30 May 2013.

8 Roger, Véronique L., Alan S. Go, Donald M. Lloyd-Jones, Emelia J. Benjamin, and Jarett D. Berry. "Heart Disease and Stroke Statistics:

A Report From the American Heart Association." Circulation 125.1 (2012). Web. 30 May 2013.

9 Beck, James, Raul Garcia, Gerardo Heiss, Pantel S. Vokonas, and Steven Offenbacher. "Periodontal Disease and Cardiovascular Disease." Journal of Periodontology Online 67.10 (1996): 1123–37. Web. 18 June 2013.

10 "Periodontal Disease Linked to Cardiovascular Disease." Perio.org. Ed. Kenneth S. Kornman. American Academy of Periodontology, 18 April 2012. Web. 18 June 2013.

11 Patton, Lauren L. "The Complexity of the Periodontal Disease— Atherosclerotic Vascular Disease Relationship and Opportunities for Interprofessional Collaboration." Cardiovascular Daily. American Heart Association, 18 April 2012. Web. 3 June 2013.

12 "Gum disease treatment can lower annual medical costs for people with heart disease and stroke." United Concordia Dental Insurance. United Concordia, 26 February 2013. Web. 5 June 2013.

13 Piconi, Stefania, Daria Trabattoni, Cristina Luraghi, Edoardo Perilli, and Manuela Borelli. "Treatment of periodontal disease results in improvements in endothelial dysfunction and reduction of the carotid intima-media thickness." PubMed Central 23.4 (2009): 1196–204. Web. 3 June 2013.

14 Sfanos, Karen S., and Angelo M. De Marzo. "Prostate cancer and inflammation: the evidence." PubMed Central 60.1 (2012): 1365– 2559. Web. 3 June 2013.

15 University of Georgia. "Low oxygen levels could drive cancer growth, research suggests." ScienceDaily, 3 May 2012. Web. 3 June 2013.

16 Soto-Barreras, Uriel, Javier O. Olvera-Rubio, Juan P. Loyola-Rodriguez, Juan F. Reyes-Macias, and Rita E. Martinez-Martinez. "Peripheral Arterial Disease Associated With Caries and Periodontal Disease." Journal of Periodontology 84.4 (2013): 486–94. Web. 3 June 2013.

17 Taylor, George W., and Wenche S. Borgnakke. "Periodontal disease: associations with diabetes, glycemic control and complications." Oral Diseases 14.3 (2008): 191–203. Web. 3 June 2013.

18 Mealey, Brian L. "Periodontal disease and diabetes: A two-way street." The Journal of the American Dental Association 137.2 (2006): 26–31. Web. 3 June 2013.

19 "Periodontal Diseases." Boston Children's Hospital. Boston Children's Hospital, 2005. Web. 3 June 2013.

20 Baker, Lois. "Obesity-gum disease link found." The Reporter, 30 March 2000 [Buffalo]. Web. 3 June 2013.

21 Jeffcoat, Marjorie. "United Concordia proves immediate and multi-year medical cost savings from good oral health." UC Wellness. United Concordia, 2009. Web. 4 June 2013.

22 Angstadt, Jim. "Research from Cigna Supports Potential Association between Treated Gum Disease and Reduced Medical Costs for People with Diabetes." Cigna, 29 March 2011. Web. 4 June 2013.

23 Scannapieco, Frank A. "Potential Associations Between Chronic Respiratory Disease and Periodontal Disease: Analysis of National Health and Nutrition Examination Survey III." Journal of Periodontology 72.1 (2001): 50–56. Web. 3 June 2013.

24 Scannapieco, Frank A., Renee B. Bush, and Susanna Paju. "Associations Between Periodontal Disease and Risk for Nosocomial Bacterial Pneumonia and Chronic Obstructive Pulmonary Disease. A Systematic Review." Journal of Periodontology Online 8.1 (2003): 54–69. Web. 18 June 2013.

25 Bobetsis, Yiorgos A., Silvana P. Barros, and Steven Offenbacher. "Exploring the relationship between periodontal disease and pregnancy complications." The Journal of the American Dental Association 137.2 (2006): 7–13. Web. 4 June 2013.

26 "New Study Shows Gum Disease Can Extend The Time That It Takes For A Woman To Become Pregnant." Medical News Today. MediLexicon, Intl., 8 July 2011. Web. 4 June 2013.

27 Mamula, Kris B. "Study: Gum disease related to medical costs." Pittsburg Business Times (2014). Web. 3 June 2013.

28 Söder, B., M. Yakob, J.H. Meurman, L.C. Andersson, and B. Klinge. "Periodontal disease may associate with breast cancer." PubMed Central 127.2 (2011): 497–502. Web. 18 June 2013.

29 Mercado, F.B., R.I. Marshall, A.C. Klestov, and P.M. Bartold. "Relationship Between Rheumatoid Arthritis and Periodontitis." Journal of Periodontology 72.6 (2001): 779–87. Web. 3 June 2013.

30 "Gum disease treatment can lower annual medical costs for individuals with rheumatoid arthritis and women who are pregnant." UC Wellness. Ed. Kenneth S. Kornman. United Concordia, 26 March 2013. Web. 18 June 2013.

31 Miklossy, Judith. "Alzheimer's disease—a neurospirochetosis. Analysis of the evidence following Koch's and Hill's criteria." Journal of Neuroinflammation 8.90 (2011): 1742–2094. Web. 3 June 2013.

32 "United Concordia Oral Health Study: The Results. A healthy mouth could mean thousands in medical savings." United Concordia Dental Insurance. United Concordia, 2014. Web. 3 June 2014.

33 Ide, Reiko, Tsutomu Hoshuyama, and Ken Takahashi. "The Effect of Periodontal Disease on Medical and Dental Costs in a Middle-Aged Japanese Population: A Longitudinal Worksite Study." Journal of Periodontology 78.11 (2007): 2120–26. Web. 3 June 2013.

34 "National Health Expenditures 2011 Highlights." Centers for Medicare & Medicaid Services. CMS, 2011. Web. 4 June 2013.

35 Brandini, D.A., A.L. de Sousa, C.I. Trevisan, L.A. Pinelli, and S.C. do Couto Santos. "Noncarious cervical lesions and their association with toothbrushing practices: in vivo evaluation." PubMed Central 36.6 (2011): 581–89. Web. 5 June 2013.

36 Mani, Ameet, Vinay Vadvadgi, Raju Anarthe, Rajiv Saini, and Shubhangi Mani. "A Clinical Study on Dental Air Force Home Dental Cleaning System on Adult Chronic Periodontitis Patients and its Assessment to C-Reactive Protein Levels." International Journal of Experimental Dental Science 1.1 (2012): 14–18. Web. 3 June 2013.

37 Ibid, 14–18. Web. 3 June 2013.

38 "Guide to HbA1c." Diabetes.co.uk. Ed. Benedict Jephcote and Raj Singh. N.p., 2014. Web. 3 June 2014.

39 Mani, Ameet, et al. "A Clinical Study on Dental Air Force Home Dental Cleaning System," 14–18. Web. 3 June 2013.

40 Ibid, 14–18. Web. 3 June 2013.

ADDITIONAL REFERENCES
FOR FURTHER READING

Chapter 1   The Zoo in Your Mouth

Moore, W.E.C., and Lillian V.H. Moore. "The bacteria of periodontal diseases." Periodontology 2000 5.1 (1994): 66–77. Web. 18 June 2013.

Chapter 2   The Biofilm Ecosystem

Boston University College of Engineering. "'Charitable behavior found in bacteria." ScienceDaily. (2010). Web. 16 May 2013.

Roberts, AP, and P Mullany. "Oral biofilms: a reservoir of transferable, bacterial, antimicrobial resistance." PubMed Central 8.12 (2012): 1441–50. Web. 18 June 2013.

Landers, Bill. "Oral bacteria: How many? How fast?" RDH Magazine, July 2009. Web. 18 June 2013.

Stamatova, Iva, and Jukka H. Meurman. "Probiotics: Health benefits in the mouth." American Journal of Dentistry 22 (2009): 329–38. Web. 18 June 2013.

Fuller, Dorian Q., and Emma L. Harvey. "The archaeobotany of Indian pulses: identification, processing and evidence for cultivation." Environmental Archaeology 11.2 (2006): 219–46. Web. 18 June 2013.

LeVarge, Sheree. "Exponential Population Growth." The Biology Project. The University of Arizona, December 2005. Web. 18 June 2013.

"CDC: Half of American Adults Have Periodontal Disease." Perio.org. Ed. Kenneth S. Kornman. American Academy of Periodontology, 4 September 2012. Web. 16 May 2013.

Chapter 3   Periodontal Disease and Your Body

Bobetsis, Yiorgos A., Silvana P. Barros, and Steven Offenbacher. "Exploring the relationship between periodontal disease and pregnancy complications." The Journal of the American Dental Association 137 (2006): 7–13. Web. 18 June 2013.

Iwai, T. "Periodontal bacteremia and various vascular diseases." Journal of Periodontal Research 44.6 (2099): 689–94. Web. 18 June 2013.

"Periodontal (Gum) Disease: Causes, Symptoms, and Treatments." NIDCR. National Institute of Dental and Craniofacial Research, August 2012. Web. 18 June 2013.

"Ancient teeth bacteria record disease evolution." The University of Adelaide News Archive. Ed. Alan Cooper. The University of Adelaide, 2010. Web. 16 May 2013.

Meyer, Mara S., Kaumudi Joshipura, Edward Giovannucci, and Dominique S. Michaud. "A Review of the Relationship between Tooth Loss, Periodontal Disease, and Cancer." Cancer Causes and Control 19.9 (2008): 895–907. Web. 30 May 2013.

Garcia, Raul I., Michelle M. Henshaw, and Elizabeth A. Krall. "Relationship between periodontal disease and systemic health." Periodontology 2000 252.1 (2001): 21–36. Web. 18 June 2013.

Stamatova, Iva, and Jukka H. Meurman. "Probiotics: Health benefits in the mouth." American Journal of Dentistry 22 (2009): 329–38. Web. 18 June 2013.

Pennisi, Elizabeth. "Human Genome Is Much More Than Just Genes." Science. Ed. Marcia McNutt. AAAS, 5 September 2012. Web. 18 June 2013.

University of Colorado at Boulder. "Normal bacterial makeup has huge implications for health." ScienceDaily, 13 June 2012. Web. 30 May 2013.

Robinson, Courtney J., Brendan J.M. Bohannan, and Vincent B. Young. "From Structure to Function: the Ecology of Host-Associated Microbial Communities." Microbiology and Molecular Biology Reviews 74.3 (2010): 453–76. Web. 18 June 2013.

Chapter 4   Periodontal Disease and Your Immune System

Todar, Kenneth. "Todar's Online Textbook of Bacteriology." Bacterial Defense against Specific Immune Responses. N.p., 2008. Web. 18 June 2013.

Mani, Ameet, Vinay Vadvadgi, Raju Anarthe, Rajiv Saini, and Shubhangi Mani. "A Clinical Study on Dental Air Force Home Dental Cleaning System on Adult Chronic Periodontitis Patients and its Assessment to C-Reactive Protein Levels." International Journal of Experimental Dental Science 1.1 (2012): 14–18. Web. 3 June 2013.

Patton, Lauren L. "The Complexity of the Periodontal Disease— Atherosclerotic Vascular Disease Relationship And Opportunities for Interprofessional Collaboration."

Cardiovascular Daily. American Heart Association, 18 April 2012. Web. 3 June 2013.

Chapter 5   Heart Disease and Periodontal Disease

"Heart Disease Risk Factors." Centers for Disease Control and Prevention. CDC, 26 October 2009. Web. 30 May 2013.

Spagnoli, Luigi G., Elena Conanno, Giuseppe Sangiorgi, and Alessandro Mauriello. "Role of Inflammation in Atherosclerosis." The Journal of Nuclear Medicine 48.11 (2007). Print.

Chen, Zu-Yin, Chia-Hung Chiang, Chin-Chou Huang, Chia-Min Chung, and Wan-Leong Chan. "The Association of Tooth Scaling and Decreased Cardiovascular Disease: A Nationwide Population-based Study." The American Journal of Medicine 125.6 (2012): 568–75. Web. 18 June 2013.

Williams, Ray C., and Steven Offenbacher. "Periodontal medicine: the emergence of a new branch of periodontology." Periodontology 2000 23.1 (2000): 9–12. Web. 3 June 2013.

Du Clos, Terry W. "Function of C-reactive protein." Annals of Medicine 32.4 (2000): 274–78. Web. 18 June 2013.

Libby, Peter, Paul Ridker, and Attilio Maseri. "Inflammation and Artherosclerosis." Circulation 105.9 (2002): 1135–43. Web. 3 June 2013.

"Specific protein may increase risk of blood-vessel constriction linked to gum disease." American Heart Association. American Heart Association, 18 April 2012. Web. 18 June 2013.

Chapter 6   Other Dangers Associated with Periodontal Disease

"UC Wellness Oral Health Study: Understanding the connection between good oral health and lower medical costs." UC Wellness. United Concordia, 2013. Web. 18 June 2013.

"Dental and Oral Health." Lucile Packard Children's Hospital at Stanford. Lucile Packard Children's Hospital, 2013. Web. 3 June 2013.

Vasili, Ermira, Migena Vargu, Genc Burazeri, Katerina Hysa, and Elna Cano. "Psoriasis and Diabetes." Inflammatory Diseases— Immunopathology, Clinical and Pharmacological Bases. Ed. Mahin Khatami. Rijeka, Croatia: InTech, 2012. 83–98. Web. 3 June 2013.

Keller, J.J., and H.C. Lin. "The effects of chronic periodontitis and its treatment on the subsequent risk of psoriasis." British Journal of Dermatology 167.6 (2012): 1338–44. Web. 3 June 2013.

Michaud, Dominique S., Kaumudi Joshipura, Edward Giovannucci, and Charles S. Fuchs. "A Prospective Study of Periodontal Disease and Pancreatic Cancer in US Male Health Professionals." Journal of the National Cancer Institute 99.2 (2007): 171–75. Web. 3 June 2013.

Fisher, M.A., G.W. Taylor, B.J. Shelton, K.A. Jamerson, and M. Rahman. "Periodontal disease and other nontraditional risk factors for CKD." PubMed Central 51.1 (2008): 45–52. Web. 18 June 2013.

Saini, Rajiv, Sugandha, and Santosh Saini. "The importance of oral health in kidney diseases." Letter. Saudi Journal of Kidney Diseases and Transplantation 21.6 (2010): 1151–52. Web. 3 June 2013.

Joshi, Nishant, Nabil F. Bissada, Donald Bodner, Gregory T. MacLennan, and Sena Narendran. "Associations Between Periodontal Disease and Prostate-Specific Antigen Levels in Chronic Prostatitis Patients." Journal of Periodontology 81.6 (2010): 864–69. Web. 3 June 2013.

Saini, Rajiv. "Oral health links breast cancer." Letter. Journal of Pharmacy and Bioallied Sciences 3.3 (2011): 468. Web. 3 June 2013.

Kostic, Aleksandar D., Dirk Gevers, Chandra Sekhar Pedamallu, Monia Michaud, and Fujiko Duke. "Genomic analysis identifies association of Fusobacterium with colorectal carcinoma." Genome Research 22.2 (2012): 292–98. Web. 3 June 2013.

Yaghobee, S., M. Paknejad, and A. Khorsand. "Association between Asthma and Periodontal Disease." Journal of Dentistry 5.2 (2008): 47–51. Web. 3 June 2013.

Thomas, M.S., A. Parolia, M. Kundabala, and M. Vikram. "Asthma and oral health: a review." Australian Dental Journal 55 (2010): 128–33. Web. 3 June 2013.

Cantley, M.D., D.R. Haynes, V. Marino, and P.M. Bartold. "Pre-existing periodontitis exacerbates experimental arthritis in a mouse model." PubMed Central 38.6 (2011): 532–41. Web. 3 June 2013.

Carter, Chris J. "Alzheimer's Disease: A Pathogenetic Autoimmune Disorder Caused by Herpes Simplex in a Gene-Dependent Manner." International Journal of Alzheimer's Disease 2010 (2010). Web. 3 June 2013.

Poveda Roda, Rafael, Yolanda Jiménez, Enrique Carbonell, Carmen Gavaldá, and María Margaix Muñoz. "Bacteremia originating in the oral cavity. A review." Medicina Oral Patología Oral y Cirugía Bucal 13.6 (2008): 355–62. Web. 3 June 2013.

Forner, L., T. Larsen, M. Kilian, and P. Holmstrup. "Incidence of bacteremia after chewing, tooth brushing and scaling." PubMed Central 33.6 (2006): 401–07. Web. 3 June 2013.

Bobetsis, Yiorgos A., Silvana P. Barros, and Steven Offenbacher. "Exploring the relationship between periodontal disease and pregnancy complications." The Journal of the American Dental Association 137 (2006): 7–13. Web. 18 June 2013.

Bosch, F. Xavier, M. Michele Manos, Nubia Muñoz, Mark Sherman, and Angela M. Jansen. "Prevalence of Human Papillomavirus in Cervical Cancer: a Worldwide Perspective." Journal of the National Cancer Institute 87.11 (1995): 796–802. Web. 18 June 2013.

Tjalsma, Harold, and Annemarie Boleij. "Intestinal Host-Microbiome Interactions." Colorectal Cancer Biology—From Genes to Tumor. Ed. Rajunor Ettarh. Rijeka, Croatia: InTech, 2012. Print.

Sethi, Gautam, Muthu K. Shanmugam, Lalitha Ramachandran, Alan P. Kumar, and Vinay Tergaonkar. "Multifaceted link between cancer and inflammation." Bioscience Reports 32.1 (2012): 1–15. Web. 3 June 2013.

University at Buffalo. "Bacteria From Patient's Dental Plaque Causes Ventilator-Associated Pneumonia." ScienceDaily, 27 March 2007. Web. 4 June 2013.

Simon, Harve, and David Zieve. "Pneumonia—Adults (Community Acquired)." The New York Times 26 April 2012. Web. 4 June 2013.

Saini, Rajiv, Santosh Saini, and Sugandha Sharma. "Oral Sex, Oral Health and Orogenital Infections." Journal of Global Infectious Diseases 2.1 (2010): 57–62. Web. 4 June 2013.

University Of Michigan Health System. "Men Do Not Cause Yeast Infections In Women, Study Finds." ScienceDaily, 19 December 2003. Web. 4 June 2013.

D'Souza, Gypsyamber, Yuri Agrawal, Jane Halpern, Sacared Bodison, and Maura L. Gillison. "Oral Sexual Behaviors Associated with Prevalent Oral Human Papillomavirus Infection." The Journal of Infectious Diseases 199.9 (2009): 1263–69. Web. 18 June 2013.

Sakaoka, H., T. Aomori, O. Honda, Y. Saheki, and S. Ishida. "Subtypes of herpes simplex virus type 1 in Japan: classification by restriction endonucleases and analysis of distribution." PubMed Central 152.1: 190–97. Web. 4 June 2013.

American Academy of Periodontology. "Periodontal Diseases Are Blind To Age." ScienceDaily, 12 June 2007. Web. 4 June 2013.

Academy of General Dentistry. "Effects of pregnancy on oral health." ScienceDaily, 23 November 2010. Web. 4 June 2013.

"Gum disease treatment can lower annual medical costs for individuals with rheumatoid arthritis and women who are pregnant." UC Wellness. Ed. Kenneth S. Kornman. United Concordia, 26 March 2013. Web. 18 June 2013.

Shanthi, V., A. Vanka, A. Bhambal, V. Saxena, and S. Saxena. "Association of pregnant women periodontal status to preterm and low-birth weight babies: A systemic and evidence-based review." PubMed Central 9.4 (2012): 368–80. Web. 18 June 2013.

Gomes-Filho, Isaac S., Johelle de S. Passos, Simone S. Cruz, Maria Isabel P. Vianna, and Eneida de M. M. Cerqueira. "The Association Between Postmenopausal Osteoporosis and Periodontal Disease." Journal of Periodontology 78.9 (2007): 1731–40. Web. 4 June 2013.

Jeffcoat, Marjorie K. "Safety of Oral Bisphosphonates: Controlled Studies on Alveolar Bone." The International Journal of Oral and Maxillofacial Implants 21 (2006): 349–53. Web. 18 June 2013.

Kavoussi, S.K., B.T. West, G.W. Taylor, and D.I. Lebovic. "Periodontal disease and endometriosis: analysis of the National Health and Nutrition Examination Survey." PubMed Central 91.2 (2009): 335–42. Web. 4 June 2013.

Wallace. "Clean Teeth and Male Infertility." Male Fertility Centre. Male Fertility Centre. Web. 5 June 2013.

Mkize, Vuyo. "IOL Lifestyle." Brush your teeth, be good in bed. IOL, 27 February 2013. Web. 5 June 2013.

Keller, Joseph J., Shiu-Dong Chung, and Herng-Ching Lin. "A nationwide population-based study on the association between chronic periodontitis and erectile dysfunction." Journal of Clinical Periodontology 39.6 (2012): 507–12. Web. 5 June 2013.

"Men's Sexual Health May be Linked to Periodontal Health." Perio.org. Ed. Kenneth S. Kornman. American Academy of Periodontology, 4 December 2012. Web. 5 June 2013.

"Health and Mental Health Services." Health, Mental Health and Safety Guidelines for Schools. American Academy of Pediatrics, 2012. Web. 5 June 2013.

Lee, Y., L.H. Straffon, K.B. Welch, and W.J. Loesche. "The Transmission of Anaerobic Periodontopathic Organisms." Journal of Dental Research 85.2 (2006): 182–86. Web. 5 June 2013.

American Academy of Periodontology. "Drink Green Tea For Healthy Teeth And Gums." ScienceDaily, 13 March 2009. Web. 5 June 2013.

George Washington University. "Cracking The Root Of Tooth Strength." ScienceDaily, 20 April 2009. Web. 18 June 2013.

Vehkalahti, Miira. "Occurrence of Gingival Recession in Adults." Journal of Periodontology Online 60.11 (1989): 599–603. Web. 18 June 2013.

Chapter 7   Put Your Money Where Your Mouth Is

Axelsson, P., and J. Lindhe. "Effect of controlled oral hygiene procedures on
     caries and periodontal disease in adults." Journal of Clinical
     Periodontology 5.2 (2005): 133–51. Web. 4 June 2013.

Chapter 8   Healthcare—Dental Care

Taxin, Christine. "Shift your focus: the new generation of dental billing."
     Dentistry IQ, 2011. Web. 4 June 2013.

Chapter 11   Using Dental Air Force

Vibhute, Akshay, and K.L. Vandana. "The effectiveness of manual versus
     powered toothbrushes for plaque removal and gingival health: A
     meta-analysis." Journal of Indian Society of Periodontology 16.2
     (2012): 156–60. Web. 18 June 2013.

Litonjua, Luis A., Sebastiano Andreana, Peter J. Bush, and Robert E. Cohen.
     "Toothbrushing and gingival recession." International Dental Journal
     53.2 (2003): 67–72. Web. 18 June 2013.

Chapter 12   Dental Air Force Studies

Cumming, Boyd R., and Harald Löe. "Consistency of plaque distribution in
     individuals without special home care instruction." Journal of
     Periodontal Research 8.1 (2006): 94–100. Web. 5 June 2013.

Chapter 13   Conclusion

"Stay Fit: Exercise Basics." Cleveland Clinic. Cleveland Clinical, 2011. Web.
     18 June 2013.

Rosedale, M.T., and S.M. Strauss. "Diabetes screening at the periodontal visit:
     patient and provider experiences with two screening approaches."
     International Journal of Dental Hygiene 10.4 (2012): 250–58. Web.
     18 June 2013.

Lawley, Trevor D., and Alan W. Walker. "Intestinal colonization resistance."
Immunology 138.1 (2013): 1–11. Web. 18 June 2013.

Bankhead, Charles. "High CRP Levels Predict Risk of Eye Disease." MedPage
Today. Ed. John Gever. MedPage Today, 7 February 2013. Web. 5
June 2013.

NIH/National Institute of Environmental Health Sciences. "Prenatal
inflammation linked to autism risk." ScienceDaily, 24 January 2013.
Web. 5 June 2013.

Acknowledgements

I am eternally grateful to my lifelong partner, Ann Bennett, for allowing me the time to pursue this passion for controlling periodontal disease and its systemic consequences. I would like to acknowledge my parents for their support throughout my life. Many thanks to my sister, Pia Brown—without her efforts and brutal honesty, this book would not have been written. Thanks to my brother, Perry Policicchio, for always making me laugh. My dog Baci lives up to her title as a true therapy dog. I am indebted to the invaluable research done by Dr. Rajiv Saini. I would like to thank all the individuals who helped proof and edit this book: Matthew Bennett, Alyssa Brillinger, Dan George, DDS, Myron Kukla, and Patty Smetana. And lastly, I would not have the insights about this disease without my wonderful family of staff and patients.

Biography

Dr. Piero is a 1982 graduate of the University of Detroit Mercy School of Dentistry with a family practice in Holland, Michigan. He has steadfastly placed a special emphasis on periodontal disease and restorations.

Since 1984, Dr. Piero has used his clinical experience in the development of Dental Air Force, a sophisticated personal home dental hygiene system that represents the biggest leap forward in personal hygiene and periodontal disease prevention and treatment since the invention of the modern toothbrush in 1939.

Dr. Piero developed and created Dental Air Force based on professional dental hygiene equipment that can "power wash" away plaque, remove microscopic debris from between teeth, and disrupt the biofilm that grows on teeth and produces periodontal disease. Dental Air Force has been heralded as a major advancement in home oral hygiene care that can help people of all ages prevent periodontal disease, preserve teeth, and improve overall health and longevity.

He has published articles on periodontal health related to heart disease, respiratory health, diabetes, strokes, cancer and other systemic diseases. He is the Executive Editor for Journal of Experimental Dental Science, a contributing author to Hospital Infection Control: Clinical Guidelines and an international speaker.

For more information on Dental Air Force, including product information and testimonials, visit www.dentalairforce.com.

CPSIA information can be obtained
at www.ICGtesting.com
Printed in the USA
FFOW05n0057280415